Table of Contents

The book "Diabetes" emerges as a beacon of knowledge in the vast landscape of health literature, inviting readers on a journey to comprehend the intricate web of factors that define and influence this prevalent chronic condition. From its opening pages, the reader is welcomed into a world where the delicate balance of insulin and glucose takes centre stage, unravelled by the expertise of the authors.

The introduction sets the tone for a profound exploration, emphasizing the urgency of understanding diabetes—a health challenge that touches the lives of millions globally. It beckons readers to delve into the depths of a condition that extends beyond its surface manifestations, urging them to explore the multifaceted dimensions that contribute to the development, progression, and management of diabetes.

As the curtains rise on this literary endeavour, the authors skilfully craft a narrative that not only imparts knowledge but also fosters empathy and awareness. The introduction serves as a gateway, beckoning both healthcare professionals and the general public to embark on a collective journey of discovery—one that transcends textbook definitions and embraces the human stories woven into the fabric of diabetes. This book stands as a testament to the power of understanding, offering a nuanced perspective that empowers readers to navigate the complexities of diabetes with newfound insight and compassion.

Understanding Diabetes as a Chronic Health Condition:

Diabetes is a chronic health condition characterized by elevated levels of glucose in the blood. To comprehend the gravity of this ailment, it is crucial to recognize the normal functioning of the body's intricate metabolic processes. In a healthy individual, the pancreas plays a pivotal role in maintaining blood sugar levels by producing insulin—a hormone that facilitates the uptake of glucose by cells, thereby regulating its concentration in the bloodstream.

In diabetes, however, this delicate balance is disrupted. The body either fails to produce sufficient insulin (Type 1 diabetes) or cannot effectively utilize the insulin it produces (Type 2 diabetes and gestational diabetes). This disruption leads to persistent hyperglycaemia, a condition where blood sugar levels remain elevated, contributing to a myriad of health complications.

Overview of Different Types of Diabetes:

1. Type 1 Diabetes:

Type 1 diabetes is an autoimmune condition where the body's immune system mistakenly attacks and destroys insulin-producing beta cells in the pancreas. This results in a severe insulin deficiency, necessitating lifelong insulin replacement through injections or an insulin pump. Typically diagnosed in childhood or adolescence, Type 1 diabetes requires vigilant monitoring of blood sugar levels and meticulous management of insulin doses.

2. Type 2 Diabetes:

Unlike Type 1 diabetes, Type 2 diabetes is characterized by insulin resistance—a condition where cells fail to respond adequately to insulin. Initially, the pancreas compensates by producing more insulin, but over time, it may fail to meet the body's demands. Type 2 diabetes is often linked to lifestyle factors, including sedentary behaviour, poor dietary choices, and obesity. Management involves lifestyle modifications, oral medications, and, in some cases, insulin therapy.

3. Gestational Diabetes:

Gestational diabetes occurs during pregnancy when hormonal changes lead to insulin resistance. This condition can affect both the mother and the developing foetus, increasing the risk of complications. While gestational diabetes typically resolves after childbirth, it raises the likelihood of developing Type 2 diabetes later in life for both the mother and child. Management involves blood sugar monitoring, dietary adjustments, and sometimes insulin therapy.

The Role of Insulin and Glucose in the Body:

Understanding diabetes necessitates a grasp of the intricate interplay between insulin and glucose within the body. When food is consumed, the digestive system breaks down carbohydrates into glucose—a primary source of energy for cells. In response, the pancreas releases insulin into the bloodstream, signaling cells to absorb glucose. This process ensures that cells receive the necessary fuel for their functions, maintaining blood sugar levels within a narrow range.

In Type 1 diabetes, the absence of insulin disrupts this process, leading to unchecked glucose levels. Individuals with Type 1 diabetes must carefully monitor their blood sugar and administer exogenous insulin to mimic the physiological response.

In Type 2 diabetes, insulin resistance hampers the efficient utilization of insulin by cells, resulting in elevated blood sugar levels. Over time, the pancreas may struggle to produce sufficient insulin, exacerbating the condition.

Lifestyle modifications, such as regular exercise and a balanced diet, play a pivotal role in managing Type 2 diabetes. Medications and insulin therapy may also be prescribed to enhance insulin sensitivity and regulate blood sugar.

Gestational diabetes, a temporary condition during pregnancy, requires careful monitoring to prevent complications for both mother and child. Lifestyle adjustments, monitoring blood sugar levels, and, in some cases, insulin therapy are integral components of managing gestational diabetes.

The authors meticulously dissect the intricate tapestry of signs and symptoms that herald the presence of this pervasive health condition. Through a detailed examination, the book sheds light on the importance of early detection and diagnosis, unravelling the nuanced variations in symptoms between Type 1 and Type 2 diabetes.

Common Symptoms of Diabetes:

The onset of diabetes often manifests through a constellation of symptoms that, when recognized early, can serve as crucial indicators prompting further investigation. "Diabetes" meticulously explores these symptoms, offering a comprehensive understanding of the body's distress signals.

Polyuria, or excessive urination, stands as one of the hallmark symptoms. Individuals with diabetes experience an increased frequency of urination as the kidneys work overtime to eliminate excess glucose from the bloodstream. This excessive urination can lead to dehydration, a phenomenon further explored within the book's pages.

Closely linked to polyuria is polydipsia, an unquenchable thirst. The body's attempt to compensate for fluid loss through increased urination triggers an overwhelming sense of thirst, creating a cycle that, if left unchecked, can contribute to complications such as dehydration and electrolyte imbalances.

Polyphagia, or excessive hunger, represents another pivotal symptom. Despite increased calorie intake, individuals with diabetes may experience persistent hunger due to the body's inability to effectively utilize glucose, leaving cells starved for energy.

Unexplained weight loss is a paradoxical feature often associated with diabetes. As the body resorts to breaking down muscle and fat for energy due to inadequate glucose utilization, individuals may notice significant and unintentional weight loss.

Fatigue permeates the daily lives of those with diabetes. The inefficiency in glucose metabolism hampers the body's energy production, leading to persistent fatigue and a sense of lethargy that can impact both physical and cognitive functions.

Blurred vision is a symptom intricately tied to diabetes. Elevated blood sugar levels can affect the lenses of the eyes, leading to changes in vision. "Diabetes" navigates the relationship between diabetes and ocular health, emphasizing the importance of regular eye examinations.

Importance of Early Detection and Diagnosis:

The book underscores the critical importance of early detection and diagnosis in mitigating the potentially severe consequences of diabetes.

Timely intervention can significantly improve outcomes, preventing or delaying the onset of complications such as cardiovascular disease, kidney damage, nerve disorders, and vision impairment.

Early detection allows for prompt initiation of appropriate management strategies, whether through lifestyle modifications, oral medications, or insulin therapy. The book elucidates the significance of regular health screenings, especially for individuals with risk factors such as a family history of diabetes, obesity, sedentary lifestyles, and age-related susceptibility.

Furthermore, "Diabetes" delves into the psychological and emotional dimensions of a diabetes diagnosis, acknowledging the impact it can have on an individual's mental well-being. The book guides coping strategies, fostering resilience, and seeking support from healthcare professionals, family, and peers.

Variations in Symptoms Between Type 1 and Type 2 Diabetes:

A notable contribution of "Diabetes" lies in its meticulous exploration of the distinctive symptoms characterizing Type 1 and Type 2 diabetes. While both types share commonalities, the book unveils the nuances that set them apart.

Type 1 Diabetes, often diagnosed in childhood or adolescence, is distinguished by an abrupt onset of symptoms. The immune system's misguided attack on insulin-producing beta cells leads to rapid and severe insulin deficiency. Individuals with Type 1 diabetes may experience sudden and drastic weight loss, extreme fatigue, and a state of diabetic ketoacidosis—a potentially life-threatening condition that requires immediate medical attention.

Type 2 Diabetes, on the other hand, typically develops gradually, and symptoms may be less pronounced in the early stages. The book scrutinizes the role of insulin resistance in Type 2 diabetes, emphasizing the importance of recognizing subtle signs such as persistent thirst, frequent urination, and unexplained fatigue. Additionally, it explores the impact of lifestyle factors, such as poor dietary choices and sedentary habits, on the development of Type 2 diabetes.

"Diabetes" contributes to the understanding of the heterogeneity within each diabetes type, acknowledging that individuals may experience symptoms to varying degrees. The book encourages healthcare professionals and readers alike to approach the diagnosis and management of diabetes with a holistic perspective, recognizing the diversity of experiences and tailoring interventions accordingly.

Through a detailed examination, the book underscores the importance of early detection and diagnosis, offering a nuanced exploration of variations in symptoms between Type 1 and

Type 2 diabetes. In its pages, readers find not only knowledge but also empowerment to recognize the subtle cues that demand attention, ultimately fostering a proactive approach to diabetes management and prevention.

"Diabetes" is a comprehensive book that delves into the intricate world of diabetes, a chronic condition affecting millions worldwide. The book provides an in-depth exploration of the various types of diabetes, their causes, and the contributing factors that lead to this complex and prevalent health issue.

Types of Diabetes and Their Causes:

Diabetes is broadly categorized into two main types: Type 1 and Type 2. Each type has distinct characteristics, and understanding their causes is crucial for effective management and prevention.

Type 1 Diabetes:

Type 1 diabetes is an autoimmune condition where the body's immune system mistakenly attacks and destroys insulin-producing beta cells in the pancreas. This results in little to no insulin production, leading to high blood sugar levels. The exact cause of Type 1 diabetes remains unclear, but it is believed to involve a combination of genetic and environmental factors.

Genetic predisposition plays a significant role in Type 1 diabetes. Individuals with a family history of the condition are at a higher risk. Certain genetic markers, such as specific human leukocyte antigen (HLA) types, are associated with an increased susceptibility to Type 1 diabetes.

Environmental triggers, such as viral infections, may also contribute to the development of Type 1 diabetes. Some viruses, like the enterovirus, have been linked to an increased risk of the condition. Additionally, early exposure to certain environmental factors during infancy may play a role in triggering the autoimmune response leading to Type 1 diabetes.

Type 2 Diabetes:

Type 2 diabetes is characterized by insulin resistance, where the body's cells do not respond effectively to insulin, and insufficient insulin is produced to compensate. This type of diabetes is often associated with lifestyle factors and genetics.

Genetic factors contribute significantly to the risk of Type 2 diabetes. Family history, ethnicity, and specific gene variants play a role in determining an individual's susceptibility. Certain populations, such as African Americans, Hispanic Americans, and Native Americans, have a higher predisposition to Type 2 diabetes.

Lifestyle factors, including poor diet, sedentary behavior, and obesity, are major contributors to the development of Type 2 diabetes. Consuming a diet high in refined sugars and unhealthy fats, coupled with a lack of physical activity, can lead to weight gain and insulin resistance.

In-depth Exploration of Causes and Risk Factors:

Type 1 Diabetes:

The book delves into the immune-mediated process that leads to the destruction of beta cells in Type 1 diabetes. It explores the role of genetics and the intricate interplay with environmental triggers, shedding light on the complex mechanisms that initiate the autoimmune response.

Type 2 Diabetes:

For Type 2 diabetes, the book provides a detailed examination of insulin resistance and the failure of pancreatic beta cells to meet the body's insulin demands. It emphasizes the impact of genetic factors on insulin sensitivity and secretion, offering insights into the hereditary aspects of Type 2 diabetes.

Overview of Gestational Diabetes and Its Implications:

Gestational diabetes is another facet of the diabetes spectrum that the book explores. This type of diabetes occurs during pregnancy when the body cannot produce enough insulin to meet the increased demands. The book discusses the implications of gestational diabetes for both the mother and the developing fetus.

The risk factors for gestational diabetes include maternal age, obesity, family history of diabetes, and certain ethnicities. The book addresses the importance of early detection and management to prevent complications during pregnancy and reduce the risk of Type 2 diabetes for both the mother and child in the future.

Genetic and Environmental Factors Contributing to Diabetes:

The book provides a comprehensive analysis of the interplay between genetic and environmental factors in diabetes. It explores how specific gene variants increase susceptibility to diabetes and how environmental triggers can either accelerate or mitigate the risk.

Genetic factors include variations in genes related to insulin production, glucose metabolism, and immune system function. The book elucidates the role of these genetic factors in the context of familial clustering and ethnic predisposition.

Environmental factors, such as diet, physical activity, and exposure to certain viruses, are intricately examined. The book discusses how lifestyle choices and environmental influences can either amplify or modulate genetic predisposition, shaping an individual's overall risk of developing diabetes.

Diagnostic Process for Diabetes:

Diagnosing diabetes involves a multifaceted approach, considering clinical symptoms, laboratory tests, and risk factors. The book meticulously details the diagnostic process for both Type 1 and Type 2 diabetes, emphasizing the importance of early detection for timely intervention.

1. Clinical Evaluation:

The diagnostic journey often begins with a thorough clinical evaluation. The book explains how healthcare professionals assess common symptoms such as excessive thirst, frequent urination, unexplained weight loss, and fatigue. A detailed medical history, family history, and lifestyle factors are also taken into account during this phase.

2. Blood Tests:

Laboratory tests play a pivotal role in diabetes diagnosis. The book elaborates on the significance of fasting blood glucose tests, oral glucose tolerance tests (OGTT), and haemoglobin A1c tests. It explains how elevated blood glucose levels, impaired glucose tolerance, and increased A1c levels indicate different stages of diabetes, providing healthcare providers with valuable insights into the patient's condition.

3. Autoantibody Testing for Type 1 Diabetes:

For Type 1 diabetes, the book delves into the importance of autoantibody testing. Detection of specific antibodies targeting the beta cells of the pancreas confirms the autoimmune nature of Type 1 diabetes. The book emphasizes the role of these tests in distinguishing between Type 1 and Type 2 diabetes, guiding appropriate treatment strategies.

Blood Sugar Monitoring and Interpretation of Results:

Effective diabetes management relies on continuous monitoring of blood sugar levels. The book provides a detailed exploration of various monitoring methods and the interpretation of results, empowering individuals with diabetes to take an active role in their self-care.

1. **Self-Monitoring of Blood Glucose (SMBG):**

SMBG is a cornerstone of diabetes management. The book elucidates the process of using a glucometer to measure blood glucose levels at home. It provides practical insights into optimal testing times, frequency, and the importance of maintaining a log to track patterns and identify trends.

2. **Continuous Glucose Monitoring (CGM):**

The book also introduces readers to CGM, an advanced monitoring technology that provides real-time data on glucose levels. It explains how a small sensor placed under the skin measures glucose continuously, offering a comprehensive picture of daily fluctuations. The book underscores the benefits of CGM in enhancing diabetes management and preventing complications.

3. Interpretation of Results:

Understanding blood sugar readings is crucial for making informed decisions about medication, diet, and lifestyle. The book guides readers through the interpretation of results, explaining target ranges for fasting and postprandial glucose levels. It emphasizes the importance of consulting healthcare professionals to adjust treatment plans based on individualized goals and preferences.

Importance of Regular Check-Ups and Screenings for Diabetes Management:

Regular check-ups and screenings are integral components of diabetes management. The book highlights the significance of ongoing medical supervision to prevent complications, optimize treatment plans, and address evolving health needs.

1. Routine Check-Ups:

The book stresses the importance of regular medical check-ups, where healthcare providers assess overall health, monitor blood pressure, and conduct screenings for diabetes-related complications. It explains how these check-ups provide opportunities to discuss lifestyle modifications, medication adjustments, and preventive measures.

2. Screenings for Complications:

Diabetes is associated with a range of complications affecting the eyes, kidneys, nerves, and cardiovascular system. The book details the importance of screenings for diabetic retinopathy, nephropathy, neuropathy, and cardiovascular diseases. It emphasizes how early detection enables timely intervention, preventing or mitigating the impact of these complications.

3. Patient Education and Empowerment:

The book underscores the role of patient education in fostering self-empowerment. It encourages individuals with diabetes to actively participate in their care by understanding the importance of regular check-ups and screenings. The book provides resources for accessing reliable information and fostering a sense of responsibility for one's health.

A Comprehensive Guide to Treatment Approaches

A detailed exploration of diverse treatment approaches for managing diabetes, focusing on both Type 1 and Type 2 diabetes. It comprehensively covers medications, insulin therapy, and lifestyle modifications, emphasizing the integral roles of diet, exercise, and weight management in achieving optimal diabetes control.

Overview of Various Treatment Options for Diabetes:

1. Medications:

The book meticulously outlines the array of medications available for diabetes management. For Type 2 diabetes, oral medications such as metformin, sulfonylureas, meglitinides, and DPP-4 inhibitors are discussed. The book provides insights into the mechanisms of these medications, their potential side effects, and how they work to regulate blood glucose levels.

For more advanced cases of Type 2 diabetes, the book delves into the use of injectable medications like GLP-1 receptor agonists and SGLT2 inhibitors. It emphasizes the importance of personalized treatment plans, considering factors such as individual health, coexisting conditions, and patient preferences.

For Type 1 diabetes, the book explores the necessity of insulin replacement therapy, as these individuals are unable to produce insulin. The book details the various types of insulin, including rapid-acting, short-acting, intermediate-acting, and long-acting insulins. It elucidates the principles of insulin regimens, from basal-bolus to insulin pumps, offering a comprehensive understanding of the tools available for precise diabetes management.

2. Insulin Therapy:

Insulin therapy is a cornerstone in the management of both Type 1 and Type 2 diabetes, and the book provides an in-depth exploration of its role. For Type 1 diabetes, insulin is a lifeline, and the book explains the different insulin delivery methods, including injections and insulin pumps. It highlights the significance of mimicking the body's natural insulin production to maintain stable blood glucose levels.

In the context of Type 2 diabetes, the book discusses the progression of the disease and the potential need for insulin therapy as the condition advances. It addresses the reluctance and fears some individuals may have about insulin use, offering supportive information to alleviate concerns and promote adherence to treatment plans.

3. Lifestyle Modifications:

The book emphasizes the pivotal role of lifestyle modifications in diabetes management. It explores the interconnectedness of diet, exercise, and weight management, illustrating how these factors can significantly impact blood glucose control.

The Role of Diet, Exercise, and Weight Management in Controlling Diabetes:

1. Diet:

Dietary considerations are paramount in diabetes management, and the book provides a comprehensive guide to crafting a balanced and personalized eating plan. It explores the principles of carbohydrate counting, the glycaemic index, and portion control, empowering individuals to make informed food choices.

The book discusses the benefits of a well-rounded diet rich in whole grains, fruits, vegetables, lean proteins, and healthy fats. It educates readers on the impact of food on blood glucose levels, emphasizing the importance of regular meal timing and moderation.

For those with Type 2 diabetes, the book highlights the potential benefits of weight loss through dietary modifications, shedding light on how weight management can improve insulin sensitivity and overall metabolic health.

2. Exercise:

Regular physical activity is a key component of diabetes management, and the book provides a nuanced exploration of its benefits. It explains how exercise helps lower blood glucose levels by increasing insulin sensitivity and facilitating glucose uptake by muscles.

The book outlines practical strategies for incorporating exercise into daily life, considering individual fitness levels and preferences. It discusses the diverse forms of exercise, from aerobic activities to strength training, highlighting their unique contributions to diabetes control.

Additionally, the book addresses the importance of consistency in exercise routines and the role of healthcare professionals in guiding individuals with diabetes to develop safe and effective workout plans.

3. Weight Management:

Maintaining a healthy weight is closely tied to diabetes control, especially in Type 2 diabetes. The book elucidates the impact of excess weight on insulin resistance and the metabolic complications associated with obesity.

The book provides practical advice on achieving and maintaining a healthy weight through a combination of dietary modifications and regular physical activity. It explores the concept of gradual, sustainable weight loss and the potential benefits of weight management in improving overall health outcomes for individuals with diabetes.

Is an informative book that delves into the intricacies of creating a balanced and diabetes-friendly diet. With a focus on both Type 1 and Type 2 diabetes, this guide offers comprehensive guidance on carbohydrate counting, the glycaemic index, meal planning, and nutritional considerations crucial for effective diabetes management.

Guidance on Creating a Balanced and Diabetes-Friendly Diet:

Maintaining a balanced and diabetes-friendly diet is foundational to effective diabetes management. The book provides practical guidance on constructing meals that optimize blood glucose control while promoting overall health. It emphasizes the importance of a well-rounded diet that includes a variety of nutrient-dense foods.

1. Emphasis on Whole Foods:

The book encourages readers to prioritize whole, minimally processed foods. Whole grains, fruits, vegetables, lean proteins, and healthy fats form the cornerstone of a diabetes-friendly diet. By incorporating a diverse range of nutrient-rich foods, individuals with diabetes can ensure they receive essential vitamins, minerals, and fiber necessary for overall well-being.

2. Portion Control:

Portion control is a key aspect of diabetes management, and the book provides practical strategies for monitoring portion sizes. It educates readers on recognizing appropriate serving sizes and the impact of portion control on blood glucose levels. By understanding portion sizes, individuals can better manage their caloric intake and maintain stable blood sugar levels.

3. Balanced Macronutrient Intake:

The book explores the importance of a balanced intake of macronutrients—carbohydrates, proteins, and fats. It discusses how the body processes each macronutrient and provides guidelines for achieving an optimal balance. This balanced approach helps regulate blood glucose levels and supports overall metabolic health.

The Importance of Carbohydrate Counting and Glycaemic Index:

1. Carbohydrate Counting:

Carbohydrate counting is a fundamental skill for individuals with diabetes, particularly those using insulin to manage their condition. The book offers a detailed exploration of carbohydrate counting, explaining how carbohydrates directly impact blood glucose levels.

Readers learn how to identify and quantify carbohydrates in various foods, enabling them to make informed choices about their dietary intake. The book provides practical tips for estimating carbohydrate content, reading nutrition labels, and utilizing mobile apps to facilitate accurate carbohydrate counting.

2. Glycaemic Index (GI):

The book delves into the concept of the glycaemic index, a tool that ranks foods based on their impact on blood glucose levels. It explains how low-GI foods are digested and absorbed more slowly, leading to gradual increases in blood sugar, while high-GI foods cause rapid spikes.

Understanding the glycaemic index assists individuals in making mindful food choices to better control blood glucose levels. The book provides a comprehensive list of common foods and their GI values, empowering readers to create meals that contribute to stable and controlled blood sugar levels.

Meal Planning and Nutritional Considerations for People with Diabetes:

1. Individualized Meal Plans:

Recognizing the unique needs of individuals, the book emphasizes the importance of individualized meal planning. It guides readers through the process of creating meal plans that align with their preferences, cultural considerations, and health goals. The book provides sample meal plans and encourages flexibility to accommodate diverse dietary preferences.

2. Timing and Frequency of Meals:

The book addresses the significance of meal timing and frequency in diabetes management. It discusses the benefits of spreading meals throughout the day to prevent extreme fluctuations in blood glucose levels. The book also explores the potential advantages of incorporating snacks to maintain steady energy levels.

3. Nutritional Considerations:

Nutritional considerations extend beyond carbohydrate counting and the glycaemic index. The book provides comprehensive information on other essential nutrients, including proteins, fats, vitamins, and minerals. It emphasizes the role of fibre in promoting digestive health and blood sugar control.

The book also explores dietary strategies for managing other health conditions commonly associated with diabetes, such as hypertension and dyslipidemia. By addressing the broader nutritional needs of individuals with diabetes, the book promotes holistic health and wellness.

A term that has become increasingly prevalent in today's health discourse, refers to a group of metabolic disorders characterized by elevated blood sugar levels. Managing diabetes is a multifaceted challenge, encompassing various lifestyle modifications, dietary changes, and medication. One crucial aspect of diabetes management is physical activity, a topic explored in-depth in the book "Diabetes: Physical Activity and its Impact."

- **Understanding the Impact of Exercise on Blood Sugar Levels:**

Exercise plays a pivotal role in diabetes management by influencing blood sugar levels. When engaging in physical activity, muscles require more glucose for energy, leading to increased insulin sensitivity. This heightened sensitivity allows insulin to more effectively usher glucose into cells, reducing blood sugar levels. Regular exercise can contribute to better glycaemic control, making it an essential component of diabetes management.

- **Types and Intensity of Physical Activities Suitable for Individuals with Diabetes:**

The book delves into various types and intensities of physical activities suitable for individuals with diabetes. Both aerobic exercises and resistance training offer unique benefits. Aerobic exercises, such as brisk walking, cycling, and swimming, enhance cardiovascular health and improve insulin sensitivity. On the other hand, resistance training, involving activities like weightlifting, helps build muscle mass, contributing to long-term glucose management.

The intensity of physical activity is a critical consideration. High-intensity exercises can lead to rapid glucose utilization, requiring individuals to monitor their blood sugar levels closely. Moderate-intensity activities, such as brisk walking or cycling, are generally well-tolerated and sustainable for most individuals with diabetes. The book provides detailed guidance on tailoring exercise plans to individual preferences, health status, and diabetes type.

- **Incorporating Regular Exercise into a Diabetes Management Plan:**

The book emphasizes the importance of seamlessly integrating regular exercise into a comprehensive diabetes management plan. It offers practical strategies to overcome common barriers to physical activity, such as time constraints and motivational challenges. Setting realistic goals, creating a personalized exercise routine, and incorporating enjoyable activities are key aspects explored in the book.

Moreover, the book addresses the importance of consultation with healthcare professionals before embarking on a new exercise regimen. Understanding individual health conditions, medication effects, and potential complications is crucial to designing a safe and effective exercise plan. The book provides a guide on how to communicate with healthcare providers to ensure that the exercise plan aligns with the overall diabetes management strategy.

- **Benefits Beyond Blood Sugar Control:**

Beyond its impact on blood sugar levels, the book delves into the broader health benefits of regular exercise for individuals with diabetes. Weight management, improved cardiovascular health, and enhanced mental well-being are among the positive outcomes discussed. The book emphasizes the holistic approach to diabetes management, positioning physical activity as a cornerstone for overall health improvement.

Additionally, the book explores the potential of exercise in preventing or mitigating diabetes-related complications, such as cardiovascular diseases and neuropathy. By addressing the underlying factors contributing to these complications, regular physical activity becomes a proactive measure in safeguarding long-term health for individuals with diabetes.

The importance of seamlessly incorporating regular exercise into a diabetes management plan is underscored throughout the book. It not only highlights the benefits of exercise on blood sugar control but also emphasizes the broader health advantages, positioning physical activity as a fundamental component of a holistic approach to diabetes care. As our understanding of diabetes continues to evolve, this book provides a valuable resource for individuals seeking to navigate the complexities of diabetes management through the lens of physical activity.

A comprehensive exploration of the complications associated with this prevalent metabolic disorder serves as a valuable resource for individuals living with diabetes, healthcare professionals, and anyone seeking a deeper understanding of the condition. The book delves into the multifaceted complications that can arise from diabetes, focusing on cardiovascular issues, neuropathy, retinopathy, and kidney disease. Additionally, it provides essential strategies for both the prevention and management of these complications.

Cardiovascular Complications:

One of the primary complications of diabetes is its profound impact on the cardiovascular system. Individuals with diabetes have an increased risk of heart disease, including coronary artery disease, heart failure, and stroke. The elevated levels of glucose in the blood contribute to the development of atherosclerosis, a condition characterized by the buildup of fatty deposits in the arteries. This process can lead to compromised blood flow, increasing the likelihood of cardiovascular events.

The book emphasizes the importance of managing blood glucose levels through lifestyle modifications and medication adherence to mitigate the risk of cardiovascular complications. Regular exercise, a heart-healthy diet, and medications such as statins may be recommended to control cholesterol levels and blood pressure, reducing the strain on the cardiovascular system.

Neuropathic Complications:

Diabetes-induced neuropathy is another critical aspect explored in the book. Neuropathy refers to nerve damage that can manifest in various forms, such as peripheral neuropathy affecting the extremities and autonomic neuropathy impacting internal organs. Patients often experience symptoms like numbness, tingling, and pain in the affected areas.

The book provides insights into preventative measures, such as maintaining optimal blood glucose levels and regular foot care, as well as symptomatic management techniques. Medications targeting nerve pain, physical therapy, and lifestyle adjustments play a crucial role in mitigating neuropathic complications.

Retinopathic Complications:

Diabetic retinopathy is a sight-threatening complication that arises due to damage to the blood vessels in the retina. The book elucidates the mechanisms behind retinopathy, emphasizing the need for regular eye examinations to detect and manage the condition early on. Tight control of blood sugar levels, blood pressure, and cholesterol is paramount in preventing the progression of diabetic retinopathy.

Advanced treatments, including laser therapy and intravitreal injections, are discussed as effective interventions. The book underscores the importance of patient education regarding the significance of routine eye exams and the potential impact of diabetes on vision.

Renal Complications:

Kidney disease is a prevalent complication of diabetes, with diabetes being the leading cause of chronic kidney disease. The book sheds light on the intricate relationship between diabetes and kidney function, explaining how elevated blood glucose levels and hypertension contribute to kidney damage over time.

Preventive measures outlined in the book encompass strict blood glucose control, blood pressure management, and lifestyle modifications such as a low-sodium diet. The importance of regular monitoring through blood and urine tests is emphasized, enabling early detection of kidney dysfunction. The book also explores advanced interventions like medications that protect the kidneys and renal replacement therapies in cases of advanced kidney disease.

Strategies for Prevention and Management:

The book culminates with a comprehensive section on strategies for the prevention and management of diabetes-related complications. Lifestyle modifications, including a well-balanced diet, regular exercise, and weight management, form the foundation of preventative measures. Medication adherence and regular medical check-ups are stressed as essential components of diabetes management.

Moreover, the book advocates for patient empowerment through education. Understanding the link between blood glucose control and complications allows individuals to take an active role in their health. The importance of a multidisciplinary approach, involving healthcare providers, dietitians, educators, and mental health professionals, is highlighted to address the diverse facets of diabetes care.

By delving into cardiovascular issues, neuropathy, retinopathy, and kidney disease, the book provides a holistic understanding of the challenges posed by diabetes. Moreover, it equips readers with practical strategies for prevention and effective management, empowering them to lead healthier lives despite the challenges posed by this prevalent metabolic disorder.

Nurturing Health: Diabetes in Children and Adolescents

"Diabetes in Children and Adolescents" is an insightful and compassionate guide that addresses the unique challenges associated with managing diabetes in paediatric populations. Tailored to the specific needs of children and adolescents, this book provides a comprehensive exploration of age-specific considerations, treatment approaches, and the pivotal roles of parents, caregivers, and schools in supporting young individuals living with diabetes.

Age-Specific Challenges:

Managing diabetes in children and adolescents presents distinctive challenges, necessitating an understanding of the physiological, psychological, and developmental aspects unique to each age group. The book meticulously examines these challenges, recognizing that the needs of a preschooler with diabetes vastly differ from those of a teenager entering adolescence.

For younger children, the emphasis is on simplifying diabetes management for both the child and the caregiver. The book delves into age-appropriate methods of blood glucose monitoring, insulin administration, and fostering a supportive environment that encourages the child's understanding of their condition without overwhelming them.

As children transition into adolescence, a myriad of hormonal and lifestyle changes add complexity to diabetes management. The book addresses issues such as insulin resistance during puberty, the impact of peer influences on self-care, and the importance of fostering independence in diabetes management while providing a safety net of support.

Treatment Approaches:

The book outlines various age-specific treatment approaches, considering the developmental stages and physiological changes that children and adolescents undergo. It explores the use of insulin pumps, continuous glucose monitoring systems, and age-appropriate insulin regimens tailored to the child's lifestyle and preferences.

Moreover, the importance of involving pediatric endocrinologists, diabetes educators, and mental health professionals is highlighted. The book advocates for a multidisciplinary approach that recognizes the interconnected nature of physical and emotional well-being, addressing not only the medical aspects of diabetes but also the psychosocial aspects that are particularly pronounced during adolescence.

Role of Parents and Caregivers:

The pivotal role of parents and caregivers in the care of children with diabetes is a central theme in the book. It delves into the emotional toll on parents, offering guidance on how to navigate the complexities of managing their child's diabetes while promoting a sense of normalcy. The book emphasizes open communication within the family, fostering an environment where the child feels supported and understood.

Practical tips for parents, such as organizing diabetes-friendly meals, managing blood glucose monitoring during sleepovers and playdates, and addressing the emotional well-being of the child, are discussed. Additionally, the book explores strategies for balancing the dual roles of caregivers and advocates for their child's diabetes care within the school environment.

Role of Schools:

Recognizing the considerable amount of time children spend in school, the book underscores the importance of collaboration between parents, healthcare providers, and school personnel. It explores strategies for creating diabetes-friendly school environments, including training teachers and staff to recognize and respond to diabetes emergencies, establishing structured meal plans, and allowing flexibility for blood glucose monitoring and insulin administration.

Moreover, the book advocates for fostering a supportive and inclusive atmosphere that educates classmates about diabetes, reducing stigma and creating a sense of normalcy for children with diabetes. It encourages schools to accommodate the unique needs of each child, acknowledging that diabetes management is not a one-size-fits-all approach.

By addressing age-specific challenges, treatment approaches, and the critical roles of parents, caregivers, and schools, the book serves as a comprehensive resource. It not only provides practical insights into managing the physical aspects of diabetes but also underscores the importance of addressing the emotional and social well-being of children and adolescents living with this chronic condition. In doing so, it empowers families and communities to create nurturing environments that enable children and adolescents with diabetes to thrive.

"Diabetes in Older Adults" serves as a comprehensive and empathetic guide, delving into the intricacies of managing diabetes in the elderly population. This book recognizes the unique challenges and considerations that come with aging, offering valuable insights into age-related factors influencing diabetes care. It provides a holistic approach to balancing medication, nutrition, and lifestyle considerations, aiming to promote health and well-being during the golden years.

Age-Related Factors Influencing Diabetes Care:

As individuals age, various physiological and lifestyle factors influence diabetes management. The book begins by exploring these age-related factors, acknowledging that the aging process can impact insulin sensitivity, beta-cell function, and overall glucose metabolism. It sheds light on the importance of recognizing these changes to tailor diabetes care effectively.

Moreover, the book addresses the prevalence of comorbidities in older adults, such as cardiovascular disease, osteoporosis, and cognitive decline. Understanding the interplay between diabetes and these conditions is crucial for a comprehensive approach to care. The book advocates for a patient-centered model that considers the individual's overall health, functional status, and quality of life.

Balancing Medication, Nutrition, and Lifestyle Considerations:

One of the central themes of the book revolves around achieving a delicate balance between medication, nutrition, and lifestyle considerations in older adults with diabetes. It acknowledges that medication regimens may need adjustments due to changes in kidney function and potential interactions with other medications taken for comorbid conditions.

The book delves into the importance of personalized nutrition plans, recognizing the significance of maintaining a well-balanced diet while considering factors such as dental health, chewing difficulties, and changes in appetite that often accompany aging. It explores dietary modifications to manage blood glucose levels effectively, emphasizing the role of healthcare professionals, including dietitians, in crafting individualized nutrition strategies.

Furthermore, the book encourages a holistic approach to lifestyle considerations, emphasizing the importance of physical activity tailored to the older adult's capabilities. It explores low-impact exercises, flexibility routines, and the benefits of maintaining muscle mass to support overall health. The book underscores the role of mental and emotional well-being, advocating for activities that enhance cognitive function and reduce stress.

Medication Management:

The book provides a nuanced exploration of medication management in older adults with diabetes. It recognizes that older adults may be more vulnerable to medication side effects and interactions, necessitating a careful and individualized approach. The book explores the potential benefits of simplifying medication regimens, considering the impact of polypharmacy on adherence and overall well-being.

The importance of regular medication reviews with healthcare providers is emphasized, ensuring that the benefits of diabetes medications outweigh potential risks. Additionally, the book discusses advancements in diabetes management, such as the use of newer medications with favourable safety profiles for older adults.

Preventive Care and Screening:

Preventive care and screening are paramount in the care of older adults with diabetes. The book advocates for regular health check-ups, including eye exams, foot examinations, and cardiovascular assessments. It explores the importance of immunizations and screenings for complications such as neuropathy and nephropathy.

The book also addresses the significance of early detection and management of hypoglycaemia, a common concern in older adults, and educates both healthcare providers and patients on recognizing warning signs and implementing preventive measures.

Quality of Life and End-of-Life Considerations:

Recognizing the broader context of care in older adults with diabetes, the book explores the concept of quality of life and end-of-life considerations. It encourages open communication between healthcare providers, patients, and their families regarding treatment goals, preferences, and expectations.

The book discusses the role of advance care planning, palliative care, and hospice care in providing comprehensive support for older adults with diabetes nearing the end of life. It emphasizes the importance of maintaining dignity, autonomy, and a sense of purpose in the later stages of life, acknowledging that diabetes care should align with an individual's values and preferences.

By addressing age-related factors influencing diabetes care and promoting a balanced approach to medication, nutrition, and lifestyle considerations, the book empowers older adults to lead healthy and fulfilling lives. It serves as a testament to the idea that with tailored and compassionate care, individuals with diabetes can age gracefully, maintaining their well-being and enjoying their golden years with vitality and resilience.

Emotional Well-being and Diabetes is a groundbreaking exploration into the often-overlooked dimension of living with diabetes—the psychological impact. This insightful book dives deep into the intricate relationship between diabetes and emotional health, shedding light on the challenges of coping with stress, anxiety, and depression associated with the condition. It advocates for a holistic approach to diabetes care, recognizing that emotional well-being is integral to achieving comprehensive and effective management.

Psychological Impact of Living with Diabetes:

The book begins by delving into the profound psychological impact of living with diabetes, recognizing that this chronic condition extends beyond its physical manifestations. The constant vigilance required for blood glucose monitoring, medication management, and lifestyle adjustments can contribute to feelings of overwhelm, frustration, and even guilt.

Individuals with diabetes often face unique stressors, ranging from the fear of hypoglycaemia to the long-term implications of complications. The book explores the emotional toll of diabetes, acknowledging the anxiety associated with the unpredictability of blood glucose levels and the potential for acute and chronic complications. It emphasizes the importance of validating these emotions and fostering an open dialogue to address the psychological burden that diabetes can impose.

Coping with Stress, Anxiety, and Depression:

Recognizing the prevalence of stress, anxiety, and depression in individuals with diabetes, the book provides a nuanced examination of coping strategies. It acknowledges that the emotional impact of diabetes is multifaceted, influenced by factors such as age, gender, cultural background, and individual resilience.

The book explores mindfulness and stress-reduction techniques, emphasizing their potential to mitigate the psychological burden of diabetes. Mindfulness practices, including meditation and deep-breathing exercises, are presented as valuable tools for cultivating a sense of calm and promoting emotional well-being.

Additionally, the book discusses the importance of building a robust support system, involving healthcare providers, family, friends, and diabetes support groups. Social connections play a vital role in providing emotional support, reducing feelings of isolation, and fostering a sense of community among individuals facing similar challenges.

Moreover, the book addresses the intersection between diabetes and mental health conditions such as anxiety and depression. It highlights the need for integrated care that addresses both the physical and emotional aspects of diabetes. Collaborative efforts between endocrinologists, mental health professionals, and diabetes educators are essential in providing comprehensive care for individuals dealing with both diabetes and mental health challenges.

The Importance of a Holistic Approach to Diabetes Care:

Central to the book's theme is the advocacy for a holistic approach to diabetes care—one that recognizes the inseparable connection between physical and emotional well-being. The book underscores that successful diabetes management goes beyond blood glucose control and medication adherence; it encompasses the overall quality of life and emotional resilience of individuals with diabetes.

The holistic approach encourages healthcare providers to consider the psychosocial aspects of diabetes during clinical encounters. It involves incorporating routine screenings for emotional well-being, providing resources for mental health support, and fostering an open and non-judgmental communication style that encourages patients to share their emotional experiences.

Furthermore, the book explores the role of education in empowering individuals with diabetes to navigate the emotional landscape of their condition. Educating patients about the psychological impact of diabetes, normalizing their emotional responses, and equipping them with coping strategies fosters a proactive and resilient mindset.

The book advocates for the integration of mental health professionals into diabetes care teams. Psychologists and counselors play a crucial role in providing targeted support, addressing specific concerns related to stress, anxiety, and depression, and collaborating with other healthcare providers to ensure a comprehensive and coordinated approach.

By exploring the psychological impact of living with diabetes and offering practical strategies for coping with stress, anxiety, and depression, the book serves as a beacon of support for individuals, caregivers, and healthcare professionals alike.

The advocacy for a holistic approach to diabetes care is a transformative paradigm shift that acknowledges the interconnected nature of physical and emotional well-being. Through fostering open communication, building robust support systems, and integrating mental health into diabetes care, the book inspires a new era in diabetes management—one that prioritizes not only glycaemic control but also the emotional resilience and overall quality of life of individuals living with diabetes. Ultimately, "Emotional Well-being and Diabetes" empowers individuals to navigate the emotional landscape of diabetes with grace, resilience, and a renewed sense of well-being.

This empowering guide is not just about managing the condition; it's a celebration of life, offering strategies for maintaining a high quality of life while effectively managing diabetes. Through inspiring stories of individuals thriving with diabetes, the book encourages readers to adopt a positive mindset and a proactive approach to diabetes management.

Strategies for Maintaining a High Quality of Life:

The book begins by outlining a spectrum of strategies aimed at helping individuals maintain a high quality of life while managing diabetes. It recognizes that the key to successful diabetes management lies not just in glycemic control but in embracing a holistic approach that addresses physical, emotional, and social well-being.

1. **Education and Empowerment:** Central to living well with diabetes is knowledge. The book advocates for continuous education about the condition, ensuring that individuals have a deep understanding of their treatment options, lifestyle modifications, and the importance of regular monitoring. Empowering individuals with the tools and information they need fosters a sense of control and self-efficacy.

2. **Healthy Lifestyle Choices:** The book explores the significance of adopting and maintaining a healthy lifestyle. From a balanced diet that aligns with diabetes management to regular physical activity that promotes overall well-being, these choices are fundamental to living well with diabetes. The book provides practical tips on meal planning, exercise routines, and stress reduction techniques that contribute to a healthier lifestyle.

3. **Effective Medication Management:** The book emphasizes the importance of medication adherence and collaboration with healthcare providers to fine-tune treatment plans. By finding the right balance between medication, dosage, and timing, individuals can optimize glycaemic control and minimize the impact of diabetes on daily life.

Inspiring Stories of Individuals Thriving with Diabetes:

A hallmark of "Living Well with Diabetes" is the inclusion of inspiring stories that showcase the resilience and triumph of individuals thriving with diabetes. These narratives provide real-world examples of how individuals have turned challenges into opportunities and embraced a positive, fulfilling life despite the presence of diabetes.

These stories highlight the diversity of experiences within the diabetes community, demonstrating that there is no one-size-fits-all approach to living well with the condition. From athletes achieving remarkable feats to artists expressing their creativity, these narratives dispel myths and stereotypes about diabetes, proving that a diagnosis does not define a person's capabilities or potential.

The book weaves these stories into the fabric of its message, illustrating that a positive mindset, coupled with effective diabetes management, can unlock a world of possibilities. By showcasing resilience, determination, and the pursuit of passions, these stories serve as a source of inspiration for readers facing similar challenges.

Encouragement for Adopting a Positive Mindset:

A pivotal aspect of "Living Well with Diabetes" is the encouragement it provides for adopting a positive mindset in the face of diabetes. The book acknowledges the emotional toll that living with a chronic condition can take and emphasizes the importance of cultivating a resilient and optimistic outlook.

1. **Mindfulness and Emotional Well-being:** The book explores mindfulness techniques and practices that contribute to emotional well-being. Mindfulness, including meditation and gratitude exercises, can help individuals navigate stress, anxiety, and the emotional complexities associated with diabetes. By fostering a positive relationship with one's thoughts and emotions, individuals can enhance their overall quality of life.

2. **Community and Support Networks:** Recognizing the power of community, the book advocates for the importance of building support networks. Whether through local diabetes support groups, online communities, or connections with healthcare professionals, the book highlights the value of sharing experiences, gaining insights, and

receiving encouragement from others who understand the journey.

3. **Setting Realistic Goals:** The book encourages individuals to set realistic and achievable goals, celebrating small victories along the way. By focusing on progress rather than perfection, individuals can maintain a positive mindset and build confidence in their ability to manage diabetes effectively.

Proactive Approach to Diabetes Management:

"Living Well with Diabetes" champions a proactive approach to diabetes management, empowering individuals to take charge of their health and well-being. This proactive stance involves not only reacting to the challenges presented by diabetes but also actively seeking opportunities for growth, learning, and positive change.

1. **Regular Monitoring and Self-Care:** The book underscores the importance of

regular monitoring of blood glucose levels and consistent self-care practices. By staying attuned to changes in their bodies and proactively managing their health, individuals can intervene early, preventing potential complications and maintaining optimal well-being.

2. **Advocacy and Self-Advocacy:** The book encourages individuals to become advocates for themselves and their diabetes care. This includes actively participating in healthcare decisions, communicating openly with healthcare providers, and staying informed about advancements in diabetes management. Advocacy empowers individuals to shape their care plans and ensure that their unique needs are met.

3. **Lifelong Learning:** Recognizing that diabetes management is an ongoing journey, the book emphasizes the importance of lifelong learning. Staying informed about new research,

technologies, and strategies enables individuals to adapt their approaches to diabetes management, continually improving and optimizing their quality of life.

It's a celebration of resilience, empowerment, and the potential for a fulfilling life. By offering strategies for maintaining a high quality of life, sharing inspiring stories of triumph, encouraging a positive mindset, and advocating for a proactive approach to diabetes management, the book provides a roadmap for individuals to navigate their journey with confidence and optimism.

This empowering resource challenges preconceived notions about living with diabetes, reshaping the narrative to one of possibility, growth, and well-being. As readers embark on their paths toward living well with diabetes, they are invited to embrace not only the practical aspects of management but also the rich tapestry of life's experiences, knowing that thriving is not only possible but a natural outcome of a positive and proactive approach to diabetes care.

Authored by leading experts in the field, the book seamlessly weaves together medical insights, personal narratives, and socio-economic perspectives, offering readers a nuanced understanding of diabetes and its far-reaching implications.

In its conclusion, the book emphasizes the urgent need for a holistic approach to diabetes management, encompassing medical advancements, lifestyle interventions, and societal awareness. It underscores the importance of ongoing research to unravel the complexities of diabetes, aiming for more effective prevention and treatment strategies. The authors advocate for a collaborative effort involving healthcare professionals, policymakers, and the community to address the rising prevalence of diabetes worldwide.

Furthermore, the conclusion delves into the emotional and psychological aspects of living with diabetes, shedding light on the challenges individuals face daily. It calls for increased empathy and support systems to enhance the quality of life for those affected. By intertwining scientific rigor with a compassionate narrative, the book's conclusion catalyses fostering a global commitment to diabetes care, prevention, and advocacy.

In essence, "Diabetes" not only informs readers about the intricacies of the condition but also inspires a collective responsibility to confront the diabetes epidemic, making it a pivotal resource for healthcare professionals, researchers, and anyone seeking a deeper understanding of this pervasive health issue.